JOCELYN KENMURE

Love Hacks: How to Stay Connected Through Infertility

To my beloved wife, the anchor of my soul,
I've found a love both fierce and bold.
Through trials and tribulations you've made me whole,
A loving hand to have and hold.

For over a decade, you've sailed by my side
Navigating waters both calm and rough.
Through every tide, you've been my guide,
Your love, my compass sure enough.

Now upon the calm shoreline, complete,
With triple blessings, our family's fleet.
Your bravery, a tale I'll oft repeat,
A beacon in the dark, our love's heartbeat

Contents

1

Introduction

At best, the curse of infertility can feel like karma playing a cruel trick. At worst, it can feel like a thousand shards of glass digging deeper into your heart with each new pregnancy announcement you stumble upon on social media. Like a modern version of Jekyll and Hyde, the exciting and hopeful version of yourself is quickly turned into an envious green monster, wondering what your friends did to deserve their second, third or fourth bundle of joy, while you struggle month after month with the disappointing news of another failed attempt. For couples facing this daunting reality, even the strongest can find themselves drowning in emotional turmoil, uncertainty and ongoing challenges.

The harsh reality, according to sources like the World Health Organization, is that in 2023 approximately 1 out of every 6 people globally struggle with some form of infertility. This is roughly 17% of the adult population (World Health Organization, 2023). In the grand scheme of things that doesn't feel like a terribly large number, yet somehow day after day it seems like everyone around you is able to get pregnant, even those who weren't trying or didn't plan on having children at all. Infertility, or the inability to successfully get pregnant after 12 months of unprotected sex has always been seen as a woman's issue, historically speaking. This is probably due to the undeniable fact that women's fertility starts to decline as they age into their 30s. In actuality, infertility in men contributes to approximately 40-50% of total infertility cases, making this very much an issue that doesn't discriminate (Kumar & Singh, 2015). More accurate reports done around the world show infertility continuing to rise, yet prevention and viable solutions remain underfunded, inaccessible and scorned with social stigma.

When the road to parenthood is muddled with setback after setback, life as you know it and life as you dreamed it feels forever out of reach. The generic phrases said by supportive loved ones trying to fill the awkward silence like, "just relax," or "it'll happen when you least expect it," sting just as much as having to bite your tongue and refrain from the intrusive replies you're expected to keep to yourself. But the truth is, infertility is hard… on SO many levels (physically, emotionally, socially, financially). Expecting all that comes with infertility not to change a marriage or meaningful relationships may be the biggest disservice society has put on humanity to date.

Yet through the cyclical pain and longing, there's not only fleeting glimmers of hope, but opportunities to strengthen the foundation of love, trust, and support that started this journey to begin with. It is true infertility puts a couple's love and dedication to the test, but it also offers the chance to bond, rely on each other for support, and build resilience through the perseverance of adversity, *together*. In the darkest of circumstances, that unbreakable connection becomes an anchor holding you steady while navigating the rough waters of infertility. And that is what this book is all about.

Throughout these pages I hope to create a safe place to delve into the transformative power of love, offering insights, strategies, and encouragement for couples to forge a bond that not only withstands the trials of infertility but emerges stronger and more resilient than ever before.

2

Navigating Treatment Options

So you've been trying to get pregnant for about a year with no luck…. Now what? There are so many different treatment options, and everyone you ask will surely have their own opinion. Between the unforeseen expenses, side effects of certain medications, precise timing of ovulation, the twists and turns of infertility can feel endless. For years, living in a constant state of fear, anxiety and heartache became my new normal. Were we on the best path for our situation or were we just wasting more time? It felt impossible to know. Our friends and family had the best intentions of trying to help, but it felt like they never truly understood what it was like to walk this barren path. I found myself many times worrying about hiding my own feelings to over compensate for the feelings of everyone around me. No one knew what to say or how to help.

Naturally, I wanted to start by telling you some things that I wish others would have told me.

- It's okay to feel overwhelmed.
- There's no one-size-fits-all solution.
- It's okay to change course (as many times as you need).
- Surround yourself with as much support as you can (whatever that looks like for you).
- Setting boundaries to protect your emotional well-being doesn't make you a villain.
- You are not undeserving.
- You are stronger than you think.
- Don't forget about the things you loved to do before fertility consumed you.

When the thing you've wanted so badly is still not happening, it's easy to question everything. This can quickly turn into a wicked spiral leaving you staring at your partner like a stranger, or even worse, looking into the mirror to find a shell of the person you once were. Reminding yourself of the points above, as often as you need, can help strengthen the warrior-like mindset needed to get through infertility. In addition, below are tips to help navigate the turbulent waves of infertility.

Tips to Navigate Fertility Treatment Options:

Educate Yourself:

This is probably one of the most helpful and most challenging tips, that's why it's first. We as a society are lucky enough to have unlimited information at our fingertips, but it can quickly become overwhelming when there is so much information out there that is, at times, contradictory. The nuanced complexities of infertility also make it difficult to know which treatment option is the best fit for your specific situation (a lot of factors need to be considered). In actuality educating yourself is probably something you'll continually do throughout the entirety of your journey. If you are anything like me, you may even find comfort in learning more about what's available, deciphering the million acronyms associated with fertility, common side effects and current research. If this already feels overwhelming, having a general understanding of the most common assisted reproductive technologies (ART) and treatment options out there is a good place to start..

Most people have heard of in vitro fertilization (IVF) because it is a treatment option with one of the highest success rates, over 40% in some cases (Stanek, 2024). For those who don't know, IVF involves removing eggs from the woman's ovaries and fertilizing them with sperm in a lab dish. If the fertilized eggs are viable they turn into embryos which are then implanted into the woman's uterus in the hopes that it will lead to a healthy pregnancy. Even though IVF can be used for many different fertility issues, like blocked Fallopian tubes, low sperm count, or unexplained infertility, the out of pocket costs make it inaccessible for many (although more insurance companies are beginning to help cover the costs associated).

Another common treatment for infertility, and one that I have had the most experience with is, Intrauterine Insemination (IUI). During this process, sperm is first collected and "washed" in a lab to separate the healthy, motile sperm from the rest. Then, the concentrated sperm sample is inserted into the woman's uterus through a thin, flexible catheter. This procedure is often used for couples with mild male factor, unexplained, or cervical factor infertility. By placing the sperm closer to the Fallopian tubes, where fertilization typically occurs, IUI can enhance the chances of sperm fertilizing the egg.

In some cases donor eggs or sperm may help achieve a successful pregnancy. In other cases medications alone may be the only thing needed. It's important to remember that treatment plans are tailored to each couple's specific needs, with the goal of achieving a successful pregnancy. That's why tip #2 is equally important.

Build Your Team of Professionals:

Start by reaching out to a regular gynecologist and explain your situation so that they can help connect you with a reproductive endocrinologist or fertility specialist. In our case we saw this stage as building our fertility team. We had our regular gyno, who could only do so much and wound up referring us to a fertility specialist. As our infertility journey continued we added two different reproductive endocrinologists and a specialty doctor to help with our diagnosis of unexplained infertility (which ultimately turned out to be endometriosis). For some of you, the intrusive nature of getting medical professionals involved may make you hesitate to move forward. In those cases it's important to remember that they can conduct thorough assessments, including medical history reviews, diagnostic tests, and evaluations, to attempt to identify the specific factors contributing to infertility. Sometimes knowing the root issue is helping you get one step closer to making your dream become reality. This is when you may be thinking, "but is all this really necessary?" That's where tip #3 comes into play.

Undergo Diagnostic Testing:

Working closely with your healthcare team to undergo diagnostic testing will be inconvenient and may even feel like overkill but in my experience, it was a missing piece to our infertility puzzle that helped us create a sense of direction in the uncharted sea of infertility. Now it wasn't a precise calculation that told us exactly what was wrong and how to fix it, at best it was a way to cross things off the list and narrow down our options for an effective treatment plan. That being said, be prepared for your fertility team to direct you straight to IVF because it is often seen as the most efficient way to a desired result, but it's never the ONLY way. After doing our own initial research and talking with our insurance providers, we knew IVF was not a feasible option for us and were up front with our medical team so that they could help us come up with other options. They did not help us at all with tip #4 and that's why I wanted to add it next.

Explore Alternative Therapies:

Consider adding non western approaches such as acupuncture, chiropractic care, natural supplements and yoga to your overall treatment plan. While these methods may not be standalone solutions, some couples find them beneficial as part of a holistic approach to fertility. As you may have already discovered, the fertility journey is not just a physical endeavor but an emotional and mental one as well. This is why we found it extremely helpful to add alternative therapies and holistic approaches to our treatment plan whenever possible.

Consider Lifestyle Changes:

Cultivating a healthy lifestyle through proper nutrition, regular exercise, and stress management can complement medical treatments and enhance overall well-being. This is one that we didn't think about for over a year of our fertility journey. In fact it wasn't until we were well into our second year of trying to conceive, feeling stuck, that we started considering even more cost-effective ways to boost our fertility. It started with things that we put into our body, like all the unhealthy food that may be preventing us from getting pregnant. And then we started to reconsider things we put on our body like deodorant, soaps, and lotions. We got very overwhelmed with the massive amount of harmful things we unknowingly came in contact with on a daily basis, but slowly we began to cut things out or find healthy alternatives and by the end of it we felt better for it, fertility aside. This tip may not be for everyone but prioritizing self care felt essential during this challenging time.

Collaborative Decision-Making:

Although there are different roles to fill, and you can even start to feel isolated or lonely, infertility is very much a couple's journey. Open communication is crucial to ensure that both individuals feel heard and supported. This may mean having a heart-to-heart with yourself first to understand where you are coming from and validate your own feelings in order to be able to share them with your partner. Discuss personal preferences, comfort levels, and emotional readiness for various treatments.

For me, being part of a same sex marriage meant there was no way around getting others involved in the conception process (with the need for donor sperm), but I didn't feel comfortable getting a whole medical team involved if we didn't have to, because it took away the connection and intimate parts of conception. So, my spouse and I agreed to try at-home insemination with known donor sperm for a year before moving on to other treatments. We knew this ultimately required a lot more work on our part (timing ovulation just right, commuting to the donor, having legally binding contracts drawn up, among other things), but it helped me feel part of the process in very meaningful ways.

There may be times when the conversation can be uncomfortable but it's important to leave no stone unturned and to frequently check in with one another as you progress through this journey together. Working together as a team, couples can make informed decisions that align with their shared values and goals. We'll talk more about effective communication strategies in the next chapter.

Discuss Finances:

Finances are a topic not many like to talk about, even married couples, but it's undeniable that infertility treatments can be expensive. As mentioned before not all procedures are covered by insurance. Openly discussing financial factors of this journey with your partner and exploring available options, such as fertility financing programs or grants can help bridge the gap from where you are to where you want to be.

Set Realistic Expectations:

It's crucial to understand that fertility treatments have varying success rates, and outcomes can be influenced by multiple factors (age, health, available resources, etc). Setting realistic expectations can help manage emotional highs and lows throughout the process. This isn't a set it and forget it type of deal either. This is something you will want to continually check-in with your partner about as circumstances change along your path. Discuss your hopes, fears, and goals for your fertility journey openly and honestly, acknowledging that the path to parenthood may not unfold exactly as planned. I was crushed after a year of trying at home did not get us pregnant. This meant we needed to go back to the drawing board and come up with a whole new plan on how to grow our family. Be prepared to adapt and adjust your expectations as needed, recognizing that resilience and flexibility are key qualities that help navigate the ups and downs of infertility with grace and perseverance.

My spouse and I planned ahead of time and agreed to 4 cycles of IUI before calling it quits, because that felt like a realistic expectation at the time. However after our third attempt, we began to re-evaluate what our financial, emotional, and physical situation was to modify what felt realistic to us in that moment and decided to try 6 IUIs in total. This is another reason why collaborative decision-making felt so important. Having each other to weigh in on thoughts and feelings felt grounding and even relieving at times. It wasn't always easy but it did always feel worth it.

Grow Support Networks:

Having a partner to hold on to in times of need can feel like a lifeline when you're otherwise lost at sea, but sometimes it can feel quite the opposite. Regardless of the ups and downs your relationship may go through, your partner shouldn't be your only line of support. It's inevitable that you and your partner will feel and need different things at the same point in this journey. Having others around to support you individually and as a couple can become an invaluable resource. Consider joining infertility support groups, both online and offline. Connecting with others who are going through similar experiences can provide emotional support, insights, and coping strategies. My spouse and I started a YouTube channel to share all the information we were learning in hopes to connect with others who were also struggling with infertility and shed light on the struggles not many want to share. Building a community of hope became a lighthouse that shone bright on our darkest nights and helped us keep going. We may have very well given up altogether without it.

Regularly Assess and Adjust:

If you feel in your gut that something isn't working, don't be afraid to change course and try something else. Just because a treatment option worked for someone you know or someone who is going through a similar thing, doesn't mean it will work for everyone. Periodically reassessing your treatment plan with your healthcare team and your partner ensures that you are always meeting the evolving needs of your intricate circumstances. Infertility treatments can be physically, emotionally, and financially taxing, so don't hesitate to take breaks when needed either. Give yourself permission to step back, recharge, and prioritize your well-being before diving back into treatment.

Remember even though you are not alone in this, navigating infertility is a dynamic and individualized process. By combining medical guidance, emotional support, and informed collaborative decision-making, couples can approach treatment options with resilience and unity, strengthening their bond on the journey to parenthood.

3

Communication Strategies

As if the physical, emotional and financial toll of infertility isn't straining enough, incorporating the intricacies of two (or more) people's feelings adds an even deeper level of complexity. There's your thoughts and feelings and their thoughts and feelings, but then there's also your feelings about their thoughts and feelings and their feelings about yours… it all gets very complicated very quickly and before you know it you might be thinking, " how did we get here?" That's where effective communication strategies can really help. The best part is you don't have to be a healed and mature adult with a degree in human behavior to be good at this, you really just have to be willing to consistently try.

Creating a safe and supportive space where both partners feel heard, valued, and respected is the foundation of effective communication. So even if you mess up, say something you regret, or forget to include your partner in on how you're feeling- going back to the goal of effective communication- is a great place to refocus and get back on track. That's because, even if it's not perfect, effective communication intentionally builds space for partners to express their feelings openly and honestly, and provide each other with much-needed emotional support and validation. But how do you get started? Below you will find the strategies that worked best for us, feel free to take what you like and tweak it to make it your own.

Effective Communication Strategies:

Seek Understanding, Not Agreement:

Infertility can sometimes cause a tidal wave of emotions, ranging from grief and frustration to guilt and anxiety, and each partner may respond to these feelings in their own unique way. Instead of expecting your partner to share your exact perspective or emotions, prioritize empathetic listening and validation of their experiences, especially when they are much different than yours. Even if you do share the same feelings it's also important to acknowledge that you and your partner could have different coping mechanisms, and emotional responses. In my experience, effective communication works best when the focus is put on trying to understand the other person instead of trying to convince them to see things your way.

This approach requires you to meet your partner where they are and sometimes that means agreeing to disagree, while acknowledging both partners' thoughts and feelings are valid. This fosters a deeper sense of connection and trust within the relationship, even amidst differing viewpoints. Instead of viewing differing perspectives as obstacles to overcome, approach them as opportunities for mutual growth and understanding.

Something that my partner and I struggled with at one point in our journey was that she would often feel hopeful and optimistic about treatment options, while I felt more overwhelmed and pessimistic about the potential outcome. We often had to learn how to hold space for both of these conflicting feelings where I didn't try to bring her down and she didn't continually try to build a sense of false hope for me. This, at times, required using some of the other strategies listed below to stay united within our adversity.

1. **Practice Empathy:**

Cultivate empathy by putting yourself in your partner's shoes and work to understand their perspective, emotions, and experiences. This will help to show compassion and validation for their feelings, even if they differ from your own. When you can understand where the person is coming from or visualize what it's like to be in their shoes, it becomes much easier to offer support and reassurance during difficult moments.

When discussing infertility-related topics with your partner, it can be extremely helpful to approach conversations without judgmental language or invalidating your partner's emotions, which can create barriers to open communication. Another part of practicing empathy can be finding ways to show love and appreciation for each other regularly. Whether through acts of kindness, words of affirmation, or physical touch, finding little ways to go out of your way to show love, even when it feels hard, can help strengthen your connection and bond amidst the challenges of infertility (more on this later).

Use "I" Statements:

"I" statements such as "I feel," "I think," and "I need" allow individuals to take ownership of their own emotions without pointing fingers or placing blame on their partner. This helps to facilitate open and honest communication by encouraging partners to share their inner thoughts and feelings in a non-confrontational manner. For example, instead of saying, "You never understand how I feel," try saying, "I feel frustrated when I don't feel understood."

Practice Active Listening:

When discussing infertility-related topics with your partner, practice active listening by giving them your full attention, maintaining eye contact, and refraining from interrupting or jumping to conclusions. Reflect back and repeat what you hear to ensure understanding and validate your partner's feelings. Reframing communication in a more constructive and non-threatening manner leads to healthy conflict resolution. Phrases like "I hear you," "I understand why you feel that way," or "I'm here for you," help to demonstrate empathy and compassion.

Share Responsibilities:

Infertility treatment can place significant demands on both partners, from medical appointments and financial obligations to emotional support and decision-making. To effectively manage the demands of treatment while maintaining a balanced partnership, it's essential to divide tasks and responsibilities equitably and communicate openly about each partner's needs, strengths, and limitations. It can also be helpful to discuss how infertility treatment may impact other areas of your lives, like work, social commitments, and personal well-being. Be honest about your limitations and boundaries, and work together to find solutions that prioritize your collective well-being. This may look a little different for everyone, but the important part is that you and your partner help each other carry the load that comes with this gut-wrenching process.

Practice Problem-Solving Together:

Approach infertility-related challenges as a team by engaging in collaborative problem-solving. Practicing problem-solving together is a cornerstone of navigating infertility-related challenges as a couple. A great place to start is by identifying the specific infertility-related challenges or concerns you're facing. This may include difficulties with fertility testing, treatment decisions, financial strains, emotional distress, or managing relationships with friends and family. Once you've identified the challenges, collaboratively brainstorming to come up with potential solutions. Encourage creativity and open-mindedness as you explore different approaches and strategies for addressing each challenge. After brainstorming potential solutions, work together to select and implement the most viable and promising options. Put these solutions into action as a team, supporting each other through the process and adapting your approach as needed based on feedback and new developments.

Celebrate Small Wins:

While infertility may bring its share of challenges and setbacks, it's important to celebrate even the smallest victories and milestones along the way. Acknowledging moments of connection, creating rituals of celebration, and practicing gratitude, help couples cultivate resilience, hope, and intimacy amidst the challenges of infertility. These practices can strengthen the bond between partners and provide solace and support.

My partner and I turned insemination day into the ritual of indulging in fantasy and letting our hopes run wild with the possibilities of what could come. Although insemination day also marked the start of the dreaded two week wait, we always made sure to kick it off with as much energy as we could muster. Even if it was only for a 24 hour period, filling the day with uplifting hope, going out to lunch and building some time just for the two of us, helped us remember why we started this journey in the first place.

Use Nonverbal Communication:

Another hard tip on this list is utilizing nonverbal communication as a tool to enhance understanding, connection, and empathy. Being attentive to cues like facial expressions, body language, and gestures can provide valuable insights into your partner's emotions, thoughts, and needs, even when they themselves find it difficult to express how they are feeling. When you observe nonverbal cues from your partner, focus on validating their feelings, even if they haven't explicitly verbalized them, and offer reassurance and support in moments of distress or vulnerability.

It's also important to be mindful of your own nonverbal cues and how they may impact your partner's perceptions and experiences. Strive to convey warmth, openness, and empathy through your own facial expressions, body language, and gestures, and avoid inadvertently sending signals of tension, defensiveness, or indifference. Self-awareness and emotional regulation can help create a supportive and nurturing atmosphere that fosters trust and understanding between you and your partner.

Schedule Regular Check-Ins:

Set aside dedicated time each week to check in with each other about your feelings, experiences, and concerns related to infertility. Use this time to share updates, express emotions, and discuss any changes or challenges you're facing in your fertility journey. This is easy to forget so committing to the same time each week can help solidify this as a routine.

My wife and I always set aside time on Fridays to check in with each other and process the week we just had. During the hardest times of our journey we even set aside time each day to check in on each other and offer support, validation, or just a safe space to vent if that was needed. It felt a little unnatural at first, especially during the slower parts of our journey where not much was changing from week to week but as we got more comfortable with it, I actually began to crave that time together and it's something we still continue to do.

Set Boundaries:

Infertility can be an emotionally charged topic, and it's essential to set boundaries around discussions to protect your emotional well-being as a couple. Agree ahead of time on when and where it's appropriate to discuss infertility-related topics and when it's off limits. It can also be beneficial to establish signals or cues to indicate when a conversation needs to be paused or redirected.

It's okay to set boundaries with friends, family, or coworkers too. Protect your emotional well-being by communicating your needs and boundaries clearly and assertively. This may even mean skipping certain events or outings where emotional triggers are bound to happen. By doing so, you can prevent discussions from becoming overwhelming or consuming your relationship.

Trying these communication strategies and keeping them top of mind during your path to parenthood may help mitigate some of the most difficult parts of this journey. But also remember, no one is perfect and these skills become stronger over time. Yes there will most certainly be instances where you don't lead with empathy or you could find yourself getting defensive, that's OK. It's never too late to take a breath, refocus and find your way back. Practice makes improvement. Prioritizing open and honest communication, will help couples strengthen their bond, navigate challenges more effectively, and emerge from the infertility journey with a deeper understanding of each other and a stronger, more resilient relationship.

4

Emotional Well-being

As months turned into years, my life with infertility began to feel like walking into a heavy gray fog, with no end in sight. Feelings of inadequacy, loss of control, and a sense of isolation only grew. At times these emotions were so strong it put a strain on many of my relationships, undermined my self-esteem, and negatively affected my overall mental health and well-being. The more financially strapped we were, the more emotionally stressed I became. The more emotionally stressed I was, the more physically out of shape I got. Like a domino effect, one aspect of my life after another came tumbling down until I didn't recognize who I was or what I was fighting for anymore. If this is what it took to have a baby, I didn't know how much I could take anymore. To go through all of this heartache, sleepless nights and turmoil felt like a never ending nightmare. And then what would happen if we did get pregnant? Then the hard part would actually begin. Test after test, treatment after treatment, with a diagnosis of unexplained infertility, I often found my mind spiraling when all I wanted to do was make it stop, but how? Where could I even begin when I barely had energy to get out of bed in the morning?

And then I remembered a quote by John Maxwell that went something like, "you can act your way into feeling long before you can feel your way into action. If you wait until you feel like doing something, you will likely never accomplish it" (2009). So no matter how awful I felt, I needed to act my way into feeling better and that is when I decided to put action into improving my emotional well-being. In essence this intentional and difficult choice not only improved my emotional well-being, individual coping skills, and resilience but it also strengthened the bond between me and my partner, fostering mutual support, empathy, and a deeper appreciation for one other. If infertility was pulling us apart, prioritizing my emotional well-being was the tether that kept us together. The trickle down effect was more powerful than I realized.

Throughout the rest of this chapter you will find tips on supporting each other emotionally, and strategies for managing stress as a couple. These suggestions have been personally expanded over time and proved to be very helpful for me and my partner, but they may not be right for everyone. The best place to start is to choose a few tips that sound the most manageable for your situation and tweak them to fit your needs. From there you can add more or create your own entirely.

Tips for Improving Emotional Well-being

Prioritize Self-Care:

It's true that infertility is a couple's journey, but in the same way that we can perceive and cope with the world much differently, we may also have different self-care needs. Encouraging and making space for each other to prioritize individual self-care activities that promote relaxation, rejuvenation, and stress relief can make a lasting impact. This may include mindfulness meditation, yoga, exercise, spending time in nature, journaling, or engaging in hobbies and interests that bring joy and fulfillment.

Some of the self-care practices I incorporated over time were journaling, morning yoga (even if it was only for 15 minutes), listening to my favorite podcast, and roller skating or skateboarding in the evening (even if it was only for 15 minutes). This combination of activities on a daily basis helped get out pent up energy, release negative thoughts and keep me present. If I found myself ruminating on the past or worrying about the future I forced myself to focus on my senses and what I could see, hear, smell, and touch in that moment. The best part in doing this for me was learning more about myself and what I needed to feel whole. It also gave me breaks throughout the day to keep my mind off things that I couldn't control. As part of my wife's self care routine she likes taking bubble baths, getting her nails done, watching crime shows, and caring for indoor plants. We made sure each of us had our own time to prioritize self-care needs and we also made time to do some things together on a weekly basis, which leads into tip #2.

Support Each Other Emotionally:

There are many different ways to support someone emotionally so I chose to focus on what worked best for me and my wife during our infertility journey. The first was making sure to encourage time for self-care and engage in activities that promote physical, emotional, and mental well-being. Offer to join your partner in self-care practices such as exercise, meditation, or relaxation techniques, or support their efforts to pursue hobbies and interests that bring them joy, whatever that may look like for them. My wife and I get recharged by being close to the water, whether that is swimming in the ocean, kayaking in a lake or even walking along the shoreline, and we made sure to find opportunities to do this together whenever possible. When we couldn't be close to the water we made sure to build in time each week to practice self-care together in other ways (even when working multiple jobs to pay for fertility treatments). Sometimes this was as simply as playing a few rounds of Mario Kart or catching up on a new documentary.

It's also extremely helpful to give practical support to your partner by going to medical appointments together if possible, administering medications, or assisting with fertility treatments in some way. Offering to divide tasks or responsibilities can lighten the emotional load and show that you're there for each other in tangible ways.

Respecting your partner's boundaries and preferences when it comes to discussing infertility-related topics is also an important aspect of supporting emotional needs. One way to do this is by checking in with them regularly to see how they're feeling and whether they're open to talking about their experiences, but also honoring their need for space or privacy when they ask for it. A personal example of this was that my wife was adamant about not taking a pregnancy test until she missed her period, where I wanted her to take a pregnancy test during the two week wait. For me it was like ripping off the band-aid but for her it was like ruining the fantasy of what could be. Although it felt like torture at times for me, I respected that she wanted to wait, so we let the packs of pregnancy tests go unused, if that meant the process would be easier for her.

Managing Stress as a Couple

This is a lot easier said than done, especially if you are someone like me who has trouble managing stress on their own. The added layer of accountability, knowing that the way I handled stress would impact my spouse's ability to manage stress and the negative impact it could have on the fertility treatment itself made the commitment to working at this a no- brainer. Of course there were times when I let the stress of the situation get the best of me and I didn't handle it in the most effective way. The important thing was that in those moments I recognized it was not how I wanted to handle the situation and course corrected it, even if it was after the fact. I am far from perfect, but I am lucky enough to have a partner who can see me trying and who actively works with me so that we can come out of it stronger. These are some strategies that worked for us:

Foster open and honest communication about your stressors,

triggers, and coping mechanisms as a couple. We made sure to discuss ways to support each other effectively and collaboratively manage stress together. Stay informed about infertility treatments, options, and resources, but be mindful of how much information you exposed yourself to (through social media, online forums or other outlets that could trigger feelings of comparison, inadequacy, or anxiety). Instead we tried harder to focus on seeking out reliable, trustworthy and comforting support, like hanging out with friends who were not in that stage of their life or who were attuned enough with our experience not to bring it up. Their friendship will forever be like the door from Titanic, keeping Rose alive when she didn't know if she would make it, the greatest lifesaver we never knew we needed.

Keep expectations in check. We had to constantly remind ourselves and each other that the fertility journey may not always go as planned, that we could do hard things, but that it was also OK to allow space for disappointment or setbacks. Focus on intimacy and connection by finding ways to stay emotionally and physically connected with each other. Engage in activities that promote closeness, such as cuddling, holding hands, or spending quality time together, and prioritize nurturing your emotional bond as a couple (more on this in the next chapter).

Be kind and compassionate towards yourself and each other as you navigate the challenges of infertility together. Offer yourselves the same understanding, kindness, and support that you would offer to a loved one facing similar challenges, and remember to be patient and gentle with yourselves during difficult times.

Practice Stress-Relief Techniques Together:

Deep breathing exercises, guided relaxation, and couples' massages are just a few ways to practice stress-relief as a couple. These activities can help you unwind, reduce tension, and cultivate a sense of calm and connection as you navigate the challenges of infertility together.

Seek Professional Support:

It's okay to seek professional support when needed. Individual therapy and/or couples' counseling can provide a safe space to explore emotions, develop coping strategies, and navigate the challenges of infertility. My partner and I attended several months of couples therapy together and not only did it help us stay connected through infertility it was transformative for our marriage. I initially thought the main role of our therapist would be a mediator to make sure we were both getting our points across but instead they showed us how to have deeper conversations that lead to more meaningful outcomes.

By prioritizing individual coping mechanisms, supporting each other emotionally, managing stress as a couple, practicing stress relief techniques and even getting professional help couples can nurture their emotional well-being and resilience as they navigate the complexities of infertility.

5

Intimacy and Connection

Although intimacy and connection play a huge part in conception, it's also a very private thing that doesn't stay private for very long when struggling with infertility. Something that is often seen as spontaneous and fun becomes calculated and controlled, to the point where some may even shut down the sexual side of themselves altogether. It might seem that heterosexual couples would be more affected by this than single individuals or same sex couples, but for many, the essence of their femininity or masculinity lies in their ability to procreate. Anyone who struggles with infertility can experience feelings of failure and negative thoughts about their sexual identity. These draining emotional feelings mixed with the physical side effects of fertility medications and financial stress of treatments are enough to crush anyone's sex drive. In fact, a Stanford study found that about 40% of women struggling with infertility also suffered from sexual problems that cause emotional distress (Jaeger-Skigen, N.D).

Despite the fact that infertility can be highly distressing, it can also present powerful opportunities for growth. The way a couple supports one another through this difficult time can determine how their relationship develops in the future. As difficult as it can sometimes be, opening up about our deepest and most vulnerable feelings, might ultimately improve the disconnect between a struggling partnership. Being supported and understood during difficult times is what binds a marriage together the most. Overcoming challenges through emotional and physical intimacy could actually strengthen a couple's bond in the long run.

For the purpose of this book, emotional intimacy is seen as the closeness, connection, and a bond that a couple shares on an emotional level. It involves feeling understood and accepted by your partner. Physical intimacy is then thought to be the closeness and connection that a couple shares on a physical level. It involves physical touch, affection, and sexual expression, which is often a wide range of activities (from holding hands and cuddling to sex). Below you will find strategies for maintaining emotional intimacy, nurturing physical intimacy, and strengthening your connection as a couple within the abyss of infertility.

Tips for Staying Connected Emotionally & Intimately:

Maintaining Emotional Intimacy:

Explore non-sexual acts of love that foster emotional connection, such as writing love letters, expressing gratitude, and offering gestures of kindness and support. Small gestures can have a big impact on nurturing emotional closeness and reinforcing your bond as a couple. One fun way to do this is by finding out each others' love language.

The term "love languages" describes the different ways people choose to express and receive love. In "The 5 Love Languages," written by Dr. Gary Chapman, there are five primary categories:

- **Words of Affirmation:** Using praise, encouragement, and verbal affirmations to show someone you love and appreciate them. A few examples could be something like, "Your strength and resilience inspire me," "I am amazed with your undying commitment," and "I am so grateful to have you in my life."
- **Acts of Service:** Expressing your love by helping them out with duties or acts like cleaning, running errands, or preparing meals. This means going above and beyond a 50/50 partnership, more like going out of your way with intention. An example of this may be, " I know you usually do the dishes but I can tell you've had a long day and decided to do them for you."
- **Giving and receiving meaningful presents**: These might be material objects or symbolic gestures that make one feel cherished. A great example of this is buying your partner something you know they want but won't buy for themselves. This doesn't have to be flashy or expensive, it's the thought behind the gift that shows you care.
- **Quality Time:** Giving your lover your whole attention and

spending quality time together makes you feel cherished and connected.

- **Physical Touch**: Experiencing affectionate physical gestures like hugs, kisses, made up handshakes, or cuddles that evoke feelings of love and connection.

Understanding your own love language as well as your partner's can enhance communication, deepen emotional intimacy, and strengthen the bond in your relationship. To find out what your and your partner's love languages are, check out the resource page at the end of this book (Nguyen, 2020).

Nurturing Physical Intimacy:

Communicate openly with your partner about your feelings and concerns, and work together to overcome any obstacles that may arise. Explore ways to reduce stress and anxiety, such as practicing relaxation techniques like lighting candles or playing soft music to create a cozy space where you can relax and connect with each other (even if it doesn't lead to sex). Remember that physical intimacy can take many forms beyond sexual intercourse, focus on finding ways to connect that feel comfortable and fulfilling for both partners.

There may be a learning curve to this but the key is to stay open and honest. Something that can help is making time to be intimate even when you're not ovulating. By doing this, you can relieve some of the stress associated with conception and concentrate on rekindling your romantic relationship with your partner. It doesn't even have to be sex. I have heard some couples taking time to make out every night. Sometimes it leads to sex and other times it doesn't, but the point is to take the time to be intimate without falling into a routine where certain behaviors signal a specific outcome. When it feels like you're just "going through the motions," deeper connection is not very likely to happen.

Remember that infertility aside, physical intimacy ebbs and flows throughout a marriage or relationship. During the fertility journey it's even more important to be patient with each other and recognize that it's okay to have moments where intimacy feels challenging. Try your best to meet each other where they are, without negatively impacting where you are emotionally and physically.

Rediscovering Intimacy:

Take the time to explore and rediscover each other's bodies, preferences, and desires in a safe and supportive environment. Experiment with new ways of connecting physically, whether it's through sensual touch, massage, or cuddling. Focus on intimacy as a journey of exploration taking the time to discover and celebrate the moments of closeness that you share as a couple. For me and my spouse, showering together naturally created the space for this. In those moments, we were able to shut out the whole world and just connect in ways we did before starting our fertility journey.

It's easy for Infertility to consume so much of your focus and energy, but it's important to stay connected beyond the challenges of infertility. Make time for activities that bring you joy and fulfillment as a couple, whether it's exploring new hobbies together, planning date nights, or simply spending quality time enjoying each other's company. Remember that your relationship is more than just infertility, and prioritizing time to nurture your connection will bring you closer together, strengthening your bond over time.

6

Building Resilience

Building resilience together is essential for couples weathering the ups and downs of the fertility journey, in order to emerge stronger as a couple. The good news is if you made it this far, you are well on your way. Many of the strategies, techniques, and tips shared this far can be used in combination with one another with the goal building a strong resilience connection with your partner through this extremely difficult journey. In this chapter, I wanted to give just a few more tips for strengthening the foundation of your relationship, embracing the journey together, and learning to grow as a couple against all odds.

Tips to Build Resilience:

Share the Burden:

Infertility can feel overwhelming at times, but sharing the burden with your partner can help lighten the load. Lean on each other for support, and remember that you're in this together as a team. Acknowledge and validate each other's experiences, and offer comfort and reassurance whenever possible.

Find Meaning and Purpose:

Infertility can challenge your sense of purpose and identity as individuals and as a couple. Take time to reflect on what this journey means to you and how it fits into your larger life goals and values. You can also find meaning and purpose in the shared experience of overcoming setbacks and grow stronger together. As difficult as this can be at times, try to always bring your focus back to the love and connection you share with your partner. Find ways to infuse joy and positivity into your journey, even amidst the difficulties of infertility. My wife and I made it a point to try new things, even when we felt a lack of energy or were in financial strife. Getting creative and resourceful helped us create some of my fondest memories.

Embrace a Growth Mindset:

With a growth mindset you are able to view challenges as opportunities for learning and growing as a couple, even through adversity. Be open to trying new strategies, seeking out resources and support, and adapting to changing circumstances along the way. Setbacks and failures are par for the course for many relationships. Looking at these challenges as learning experiences and celebrating the progress and achievements that you make together, no matter how small, can make all the difference.

Practice Gratitude:

Regularly expressing appreciation for each other and the positive aspects of your relationship is a great way to practice gratitude. This was a harder concept for me than I would like to admit but over time it did have a lasting impact on my own mental well-being, so much that I continue to practice gratitude today. I started by writing 3 things I was grateful for every day. At first they were broad or random things just to say I did it, but as I got into the habit, the more I found to be grateful for. By the end of the month I was easily able to write 4 or 5 things down a day. Take time to acknowledge and celebrate the blessings in your life, and find moments of joy and connection even on your hardest days.

Focus on Solutions, Not Blame:

Instead of placing blame or pointing fingers, focus on finding solutions to challenges as they arise. Approach problems as a team, brainstorming potential solutions together and working collaboratively to implement and evaluate them over time. For me this was putting in a constant effort to refrain from taking things personally by actively reminding myself, "we are a team." That simple phrase really helped me to put things into a more productive perspective.

Stay Connected Beyond Infertility:

Make an effort to stay connected as a couple beyond the challenges of infertility. Prioritize activities that bring you joy and fulfillment as a couple, whether it's exploring new hobbies together, planning date nights, or simply spending quality time enjoying each other's company. For me and my spouse, this looked like planning date nights with other couples who didn't have kids. We didn't have the anxiety of not knowing where the conversation would go and it was the closest way to press pause on our own struggles even if for only an hour or two. We also tried visiting places, trying new restaurants and trying new things like participating in a self-defense class. If nothing else we were creating new positive memories together to counteract the more difficult memories that weighed heavy in our hearts.

Maintain a Sense of Hope:

Hold onto hope and optimism for the future, even in the face of challenges and uncertainties. Trust that you have the strength and resilience to navigate the fertility journey together, and focus on the love and connection that sustains you as a couple. Remember that infertility is just one chapter in your story, and that there are many paths to building a family and creating a fulfilling life together. In my experience, this tip took a lot of conscious effort and my partner and I weren't always in it 50/50. There were many times along our journey where I was feeling exceptionally low and my wife had extra hope she used to pull me out of it, and vice versa. The important thing was that we knew we could count on one to lift the other up in times of need.

Celebrate Milestones Together:

Celebrate the milestones and achievements along your fertility journey as a couple, whether it's completing a round of treatment, receiving positive news from a doctor, or simply making it through a challenging day. Acknowledge and celebrate each other's resilience, strength, and courage, and find moments of joy and connection whenever possible.

Building resilience as a couple while navigating infertility is no small feat, but it is a journey that can strengthen your bond and deepen your connection for a lifetime. That's because it can be seen as a testament to the love and commitment you have for each other. Together, you possess the resilience, courage, and love needed to navigate the unpredictable waves of infertility, emerging stronger and more resilient than ever before, whatever that may look like for you.

7

Conclusion

As we come to the end of this book, I encourage you to reflect on the journey you've embarked on together as a couple navigating infertility. Look at all that you have been through already and be proud of where you are standing (even if it is nowhere near where you thought you would be). In this concluding chapter, we'll recap the key strategies discussed throughout the book in the hopes of offering encouragement for the future.

Recap of Key Strategies:

- Prioritize communication and foster open and honest dialogue with your partner.
- Find ways to lean on each other for support and validation during difficult moments.
- Cultivate trust, vulnerability, and empathy in your relationship.
- Embrace a growth mindset and view challenges as oppor-

tunities for learning and growth.

- Seek support and resources to help you navigate the challenges of infertility.
- Practice self-care and prioritize the physical, emotional, and mental well-being of both yourself and your partner.
- Celebrate milestones and achievements along the fertility journey, no matter how small.
- Maintain hope and optimism for the future, even in the face of challenges and setbacks.
- Don't lose sight of why you started this journey.

As you continue on your fertility journey, I want to offer you encouragement and support for the road ahead. Remember that there are many paths to building a family and creating a fulfilling life together. Trust in your resilience, strength, and love for each other, and know that you have the power to overcome any obstacles that come your way.

If you found this book helpful please consider leaving a review to share your thoughts and experiences with others who may be on a similar journey. Your review can help other couples struggling with infertility find support, guidance, and encouragement as they navigate their own fertility journeys. Thank you for your support, and we wish you all the best on your path to parenthood..

Most importantly, remember that you are not alone, and that there is hope and support available to you. If you are looking for more support, please feel free to follow the YouTube channel my wife and I created @Lesbi-Honest with Daniela and

Jocelyn. In sharing our unconventional journey, we hope to provide followers with educational and entertaining content to brighten even the darkest of days. Throughout our own struggles with infertility we have been committed to continuing to grow into the best versions of ourselves while fostering an environment that promotes diversity, unity and equity as a connected community.

Wishing you strength, courage, and love as you continue to build a meaningful life.

8

Resources & Citations

Jaeger-Skigen, B. (n.d.). *Sex & infertility: How to reconnect sexually during infertility.* FertilityIQ:https://www.fertilityiq.com/fertilityiq/articles/sex-and-infertility-how-to-reconnect-sexually-during-infertility

Kumar, N., & Singh, A. (2015). Trends of male factor infertility, an important cause of infertility: A review of literature. *Journal of Human Reproductive Sciences, 8*(4), 191. https://doi.org/10.4103/0974-1208.170370:https://www.ncbi.nlm.nih.gov/pmc/articles/PMC4691969/#:~:text=Of%20all%20infertility%20cases%2C%20approximately,sperm%20motility%2C%20or%20abnormal%20morphology

Maxwell, J. (2009). *A quote from How Successful People Think.* Goodreads. https://www.goodreads.com/quotes/1158022-you-can-act-your-way-into-feeling-long-before-you#:~:text=Quote%20by%20John%20C.,long%20before%20y...%E2%80%9D

Nguyen, J. (2020, October 21). *What Are The 5 Love Languages? Everything You Need To Know*. mindbodygreen RSS. https://www.mindbodygreen.com/articles/the-5-love-languages-explained

Stanek, B. (2024, January 2). *IVF success rates by age in 2024*. Forbes. https://www.forbes.com/health/family/ivf-success-rates-by-age/

World Health Organization. (2023, April 4). *1 in 6 people globally affected by infertility:* https://www.who.int/news/item/04-04-2023-1-in-6-people-globally-affected-by-infertility

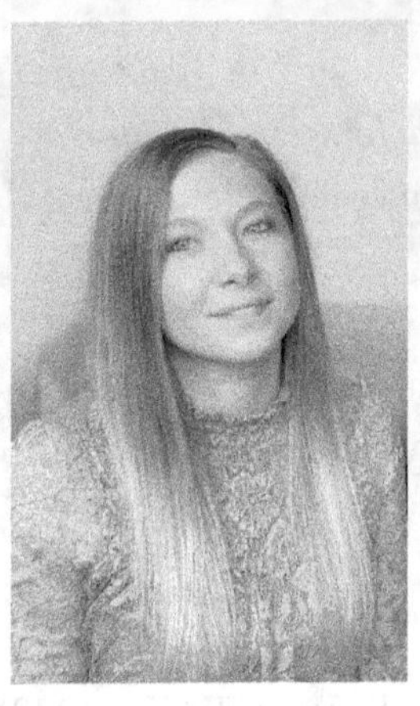

About the Author

Jocelyn Kenmure is a passionate advocate for love, resilience, and lifelong learning. With a bachelor's degree in literary analysis and a master's degree in digital marketing, her unconventional professional path is fueled by an undying curiosity of what it means to be connected in a growing digital world. Drawing from her own experience with infertility in a same-sex marriage, Jocelyn brings a compassionate, unique and empathetic perspective to her work. Her debut book, "Love Hacks: How to Stay Connected Through Infertility," is a heartfelt guide that offers practical strategies and personal insights for couples facing the emotional rollercoaster of infertility. Jocelyn's writing is characterized by its authenticity, warmth, and unwavering optimism, inspiring readers to cultivate love, resilience, and connection in the face of adversity. After years of struggling with infertility, Jocelyn and her wife welcomed triplets in August of 2023. When she's not writing, Jocelyn enjoys spending time with her family, exploring the outdoors, and sharing her experiences through social media.

You can find her on:
    YouTube @ Lesbi-Honest with Daniela and Jocelyn
    Tiktok @lesbihonest_20
    Instagram @lesbihonest_20
    Facebook @Lesbi-Honest with Daniela and Jocelyn

www.ingramcontent.com/pod-product-compliance
Lightning Source LLC
Chambersburg PA
CBHW070733260726
48660CB00007B/2816